Journey to Wellness: Anti-Inflammatory Lifestyle Guidebook and Meal Plan Recipes

Tools to Combat Chronic Inflammation and Auto-Immune Disease

1st Edition
August 19, 2024
Written by: Carey Shannon of Carolina Sunshine Wellness

Table of Contents

Dedication: **4**

The WHY Behind Our Journey: 7

How Can an Anti-Inflammatory Lifestyle Help to Combat Chronic Inflammation and Auto-Immune..10

How Our Journey Has Shaped Our Relationship with Food 11

Building a Plan-How to Shop and Stock:..13

Things to Look for When Shopping: 17

"Dirty Dozen" 12 Fruits and Vegetables that are best to buy organic 19

"The Clean 15" Fruit/Veggies Safest to Consume in Non-Organic Form 20

Staples to Keep in Your Pantry, Fridge and Freezer:....................21

Protein Options: 21

Carbohydrates:.....................22

Good Fats, Nuts and Seeds: ..22

Nut Milk 23

Cheeses to use Minimally to Sprinkle In Flavor: 23

Herbs, Spices and Condiments: 24

Natural Sweeteners:...............24

Teas: 25

Partial List of Anti-Inflammatory Foods: 25

Example List of Foods to Avoid from www.nutrition.va.gov: 28

Cooking Methods: 28

Portion Size: Easy Portioning 29

Hand Portioning: 30

Plate Portioning: Plan Your Plate 31

Tips for Eating Out 31

How to Survive the Weekends?! .36

Smoothie Recipes: 39

Blueberry Peach Smoothie 39

Oatmeal Smoothie 39

Pineapple Enzyme Smoothie 40

Berry-Watermelon Smoothie 40

Fat Burning Pineapple Smoothie
....41

Chai Vanilla Smoothie 41

Orange, Mango, Vanilla Smoothie
....42

Banana Chocolate Heaven
Smoothie.......................................42

Chocolate Dinner Smoothie......43

Mixed Berry Bliss Smoothie 44

Inflammation Buster Pina Colada
Smoothie.......................................44

Strawberry Vanilla Smoothie 45

Melon Ginger Smoothie.............45

Refreshing Turmeric Smoothie 46

Berry Basil Smoothie.................46

Green Smoothie 47

Fall Spice Smoothie (Delicious
Any Time of Year!) 47

Strawberry Peach Smoothie 48

Soup Recipes: 49

Kabocha Thai Soup 49

Cold Cantaloupe Soup 50

Breakfast Recipes: 51

Ezekiel Raisin French Toast 51

Easy Breakfast Burrito 52

Maple Pecan Quinoa.................53

Oatmeal Banana Pancakes 53

2 Egg Scramble 54

Avocado Toast 55

Spinach Egg Scramble with Berries.......................................56

Avocado and Spinach Omelet ..57

Apple, Raisin Oatmeal 58

2 Eggs, Bacon and Sourdough Toast 59

Lunch/Dinner Recipes:.................60

Anti-Inflammatory Lasagna.......60

Thai Chicken Lettuce Wraps.....61

Veggie Enchiladas 63

Quinoa Acorn Squash (p43 sp ed ce anti-inflammatory)...............65

Baked Sweet Potato and Salad.65

Avocado Toast 67

Veggie Beet Hummus Wrap 68

Unbelievable Carrot Hot Dog: ...69

Healthy Portuguese Green Soup: 71

Bacon and Avocado Sandwich with Green Salad......................73

Sandwich:.................................73

Small Green Salad: 74

Southwest Chicken Wrap.........74

Taco Tuesday 75

Lemongrass and Ginger Chicken 78

Healthy Pad Thai 80

For the sauce: 81

Toppings: 82

Chicken Pesto Avocado Boats .85

Pesto: 85

Mango Quinoa 86

White Bean Salad 87

Build Your Own Pizzas 88

Taco Lettuce Wraps 90

Anti-Inflammatory Chicken Piccata Casserole Recipe 92

Chicken Salad-Salad 94

Dressing: 94

Chicken Salad: 95

Steak Night Dinner 95

Veggie Hummus Wrap 97

Shrimp Thai Dinner 97

Delicious Lemon Pasta 99

Zoodle Shrimp Dinner 100

Easy Farro Bowl 101

Glazed Miso Salmon with Blanched Asparagus 103

Lettuce Wrap Burgers with Sweet Potato Wedges and Salad 104

Zesty Mediterranean Chicken Skillet 106

Snack Recipes: 107

Baked Sweet Potato.................107

Low Sodium Soup....................107

Veggies and Hummus 108

Garden Fresh Caprese: 109

Greek Yogurt Dip and Fresh Vegetables:...............................110

Dip Ingredients: 110

Vegetables: 110

Fresh Pineapple and Cottage Cheese: 111

Boiled Eggs and Blueberries ..111

Egg and ½ Avocado................112

Dried Fruit and Nut Mix 112

Apple and Nut Butter 113

Greek Yogurt Fruit and Chocolate Frozen Treats 114

Fresh Nuts: Almonds, Walnuts, Pecans etc 114

Small snack pack of Fresh
Mozzarella Balls 115

(Peanut Butter) Snack Balls....115

A "Date" with Mango Energy
Balls 116

Veggies and Hummus 117

Greek Yogurt Fruit Parfait.......118

Greek Yogurt and Dark Chocolate
Chips 119

Roasted Chickpeas.................119

Banana Dippers.....................120

Dark Chocolate Covered Fruit 121

Avocado Toast 121

Fruit and Almonds 122

Smoked Salmon Toast 122

Lemon Blueberry Nice Cream.124

Greek Yogurt Fruit and Chocolate
Frozen Treats 124

Carrot Juice or Carrots...........125

Dark Chocolate Cashew Clusters
....125

Lemon or Blueberry Lara Bar .126

Guacamole and Baked Corn Tortilla 126

Open Faced Rice Cake Sandwich 127

Berries and Dollop of Greek Yogurt 128

Bonus Content **129**

Dedication:

This book is dedicated to my amazing family and friends who have supported my wellness journey over the years after my diagnosis, and to all those who are faced with an auto-immune disorder or compromised health. A healthier life full of energy and joy lies ahead! I am excited for you to start the path to your wellness journey!

This book is a compilation of useful information and research that has supported my own journey to wellness after being diagnosed with an auto-immune disorder and has impacted the lives of many others over the years. It is important to note that I am not a doctor, and do not intend for this information to replace any professional medical or mental health advisement. An important part of starting the path to wellness is to take action and responsibility for your health.

Client (reader) is responsible for creating and implementing his/her own physical, mental, and emotional well-being, decisions, choices, actions, and results. As such, the Client agrees that the Coach (author) is not and will not be liable for any actions or inaction, or for any direct or indirect result of any services provided by the Coach (author). Client (reader) understands coaching is not therapy and does not substitute for therapy if needed, and does
not prevent, cure, or treat any mental disorder or medical disease.

With that being said, I am so excited that you are taking this step for you! It has changed my life!

The WHY Behind Our Journey:

My journey started years ago when I took on a new full-time job teaching 1st grade in my community with an extremely challenging group. Little did I know at the time the stress and chaos that my body would endure. I made it through the year, but as soon as summer arrived, I became ill and had many strange symptoms including extreme fatigue, joint pain, a swollen hip, and a rash on my face and breast. The doctor visits started, and they couldn't figure out what was causing these symptoms. After many attempts at different treatments, a possible inflammatory breast cancer diagnosis, and a high-dose long-term steroid regime, I was diagnosed with an autoimmune disorder.

For me, the steroid treatment was my motivation to look for alternative methods to heal my body, as I didn't ever want to take steroids again!!!

This led me to a lot of research on alternative treatment methods and ultimately to discover how nutrition, exercise, faith, meditation, sleep, and stress reduction are the key factors to repairing the body!

Over the years, I continued to work on changing my habits and began to explore changes in diet. As I progressed in my experiments, I realized that there was a definite correlation to how I was feeling. Fast forward to several years later ... I had slacked off a bit on watching what I was eating, reducing stress, etc. And not surprisingly the symptoms started to gradually return until once again, I was looking at doctor visits and medications. This brought me to the reality that this had to be a lifelong lifestyle change for me and my family! I was all in! It was time to clean out my pantry, build a plan, stock up on the right foods, prep, and start our family's journey to wellness!

I continued to support friends and family in the years to come and have seen much success! I am excited to team with you on your new wellness journey!

"Dear friend, I pray that you may enjoy good health and that all may go well with you, even as your soul is getting along well." - 3 John 1:2 NIV

How Can an Anti-Inflammatory Lifestyle Help to Combat Chronic Inflammation and Auto Immune

Chronic inflammation in the body can trigger auto-immune responses and lead to exacerbated symptoms.

Current research demonstrates that taking steps to reduce inflammation in the diet by eating anti-inflammatory foods, eliminating sugar and processed foods, increasing activity, supplementing, reducing stress, and good sleep cycles can lessen symptoms and improve overall wellness. Embracing an anti-inflammatory lifestyle can be a powerful strategy in managing chronic inflammation and auto immune. Other benefits include increased energy, promoting weight loss, eliminating bloating, and improved mood/focus.

How Our Journey Has Shaped Our Relationship with Food

Many factors influence our food choices, each shaping what we decide to eat and how we approach our relationship with food. These factors include cultural influences, health considerations, economic factors, social influences, convenience/time, environmental concerns, marketing and media, and most of all tastes and preferences, or at least what we perceive to be our preferences.

Over time we set ourselves on autopilot when it comes to our relationship with foods. It is like driving a car and arriving not remembering how you got there…or scrolling mindlessly through your phone and realizing you have just wasted 30 minutes! We go through our day eating without taking the time to enjoy the moment and be grateful for our food. When we lack awareness and gratitude for what we are consuming, we tend to make poor choices!

We also develop habits that relate our food choices to triggers that we face daily and then opt to soothe ourselves with food. Examples of triggers might be stress, life changing event, eating to soothe, relationships, low self-worth, boredom, loneliness, social events, holidays, or vacations.

I am here to encourage you to shift your journey and shape a new relationship with food! One that brings you energy and health! I am living proof that food can reduce inflammation, heal the body, and give you a new and healthy lifestyle. And did I mention this new journey includes delicious food to enjoy! **Let's get started...**

Building a Plan-How to Shop and Stock:

When building a plan and stocking up your kitchen for anti-inflammatory eating, label reading is an integral piece of the preparation! You will want to look for products that contain only real food items and are not overly processed with high amounts of preservatives. If you have trouble pronouncing the ingredients, you probably don't want to put them in your body. Stock your pantry and refrigerator with inflammation-fighting foods. The simple key factors are:

1. Eliminate processed foods,
2. Eliminate processed sugars and begin to use local honey, maple syrup, and other natural sweeteners in moderation.
3. Greatly reduce or eliminate dairy from the diet. We still utilize a small amount of fresh parmesan or feta to add flavor to dishes and eat all-natural Greek yogurt, but overall, we do not consume milk or milk products as we used to before making the change. If you seem to have reactions to dairy, then you might want to consider eliminating it for 30 days and

then adding a little back in to see if you notice inflammation.

4. Eliminate or greatly reduce gluten intake…for me this was a big one. However, I can enjoy fresh fermented sourdough! We now choose Ezekiel bread and gluten-free oats etc. Brown rice or freshly made pasta with pure semolina flour can work well for your pasta cravings!
5. Add in delicious anti-inflammatory fruits, vegetables, spices, and superfoods!!!
6. Have breakfast, lunch, dinner, and 2 snacks! **Portion size** and **types of food** are very important components!
7. Prepare! Plan to do food prep and meal planning and have fun trying new recipes!
At first, this may feel overwhelming, but you will quickly see how much better

you feel and will probably notice weight loss as well! Embrace this new opportunity to build new habits with food! Honestly, my family enjoys my cooking so much more now, and I love finding new ways to make YUMMY HEALTHY food! You don't have to deprive yourself or give up eating your favorites…you just learn how to make them in a healthier way! For example, ice cream is my favorite! I now make ice cream at home with lots of flavors to choose from using either bananas or fruit and coconut milk:). DELICIOUS! I have included a few of these recipes in the snack area of this meal plan. Try them out and let me know what you think.

MODERATION IS KEY! It is not reasonable to think that you

will start this journey and never again be able to enjoy eating out, celebrating birthdays, enjoying parties or having an occasional treat day. We all need to enjoy life! I believe that if you can honor yourself and commit to completing 28 days of this meal plan, how you feel will be your motivating factor to continue your own new journey! Each of our bodies is unique and you will start to be able to detect what triggers your inflammation.

Things to Look for When Shopping:

Protein Meats: Select high-quality grass-fed, grass-finished meats instead of factory-farmed meats. You can choose to select less popular cuts to keep the cost down.

Protein Fish: Select the wild-caught fish options over the farm raised.

Protein Plant Based: Be aware of processed foods such as fake meat replacements and stay away from these options! Opt for edamame beans, high protein vegetables, nuts or low process tofu or tempeh. Reading the labels is key when selecting your proteins.

Fruits and Veggies: When possible, choose organic fruits and vegetables and buy local farm fresh produce as they are typically grown in more nutrient-rich soil.

Gluten-Free: Plan to remove gluten from your diet and kitchen. It is helpful to be aware of foods that contain gluten, and reduce or remove from your daily intake. Some great options for bread are Ezekiel or a real sourdough bread purchased from a bakery or homemade. Also, plan to purchase whole grain gluten-free oats as they are a great ingredient to have for baking some yummy treats. ;)

Natural Sweeteners: Select a natural local honey, Pure Grade A Maple Syrup or other natural sweeteners without processed sugars

Nut Butter: Make sure to read the labels closely on nut butter. The only ingredient you want is the nut itself! Watch out for nut butter with palm oil or other processed oils!

"Dirty Dozen" 12 Fruits and Vegetables that are best to buy organic (*The Ultimate Series, The Anti-Inflammatory Guide*):

Strawberries
Kale, collard, and mustard greens
Apples
Cherries
Pears

Celery
Spinach
Nectarines
Grapes
Peaches
Bell Peppers
Tomatoes

"The Clean 15" Fruit/Veggies Safest to Consume in Non-Organic Form (*The Ultimate Series, the Anti-Inflammatory Guide*):

Avocado
Sweetcorn
Pineapple
Onions
Papayas
Frozen Peas
Egg Plant
Asparagus
Broccoli
Cabbage
Kiwis
Cauliflower
Mushrooms

Honeydew melons
Cantaloupe Melons

Staples to Keep in Your Pantry, Fridge and Freezer:

Protein Options:

It is important when selecting meat to look for local grass-fed and grass-finished meats. When purchasing fish and shellfish you should select only wild caught.
• Chicken
• Turkey
• Lean ground turkey
• Lean hamburger
• Lean steak
• Buffalo or Bison
• Tuna
• Egg whites
• Whole eggs
• White Fish
• Shrimp, Scallops or Lobster
• Full Fat cottage cheese
• Whey Protein powder

• Full Fat Greek yogurt
• Kefir

• Slow cooked whole grain oatmeal
• Lentils
• Beans (kidney, red, black, cannelloni)
• Sweet potatoes
• White potatoes
• Red potatoes
• Quinoa
• Brown rice
• Pumpkin
• Brown Rice Pasta or Homemade Pasta from Pure Semolina Flour
• Ezekiel or Sourdough bread
• Low sodium rice cakes (add nut butter and you have a quick snack on the go!)
• Hummus (preferably homemade)
See Anti-Inflammatory Partial List for Additional Ideas

Good Fats, Nuts and Seeds:

• Pecans (all nuts consumed raw and unsalted)
• Olive oil
• Almonds
• Walnuts
• Peanut butter
• Almond butter
• Avocado
• Coconut oil
• Grape seed oil
• Olives
• Flax Seed
• Hemp Seed
• Chia Seed

See Anti-Inflammatory Partial List for Additional Ideas

Nut Milks (should only contain minimal ingredients… nuts, water salt):

• Almond Milk
• Oat Milk
• Walnut Milk etc.

Cheeses to use Minimally to Sprinkle In Flavor:

• Pure Natural Mozzarella
• Pure Grated or Shaved Parmesan
• Natural Feta

Herbs, Spices and Condiments:

• Basil
• Oregano
• Mustard
• Cilantro
• Dill
• Ginger
• Garlic
• Mint
• Parsley
• Rosemary
• Tarragon
• Thyme
• Turmeric
• Cumin
• Cardamom
• Cinnamon
• Cayenne Pepper

- Local Natural Honey
- Pure Grade A Maple Syrup
- Pure Agave
- Stevia
- Yacon

Choose all-natural teas that are mostly decaffeinated. Coffee can also be consumed in small amounts, but you do not want to consume large amounts of caffeine. See the Superfood Coffee Recipe to make your cup pack an anti-inflammatory punch!

Partial List of Anti-Inflammatory Foods:

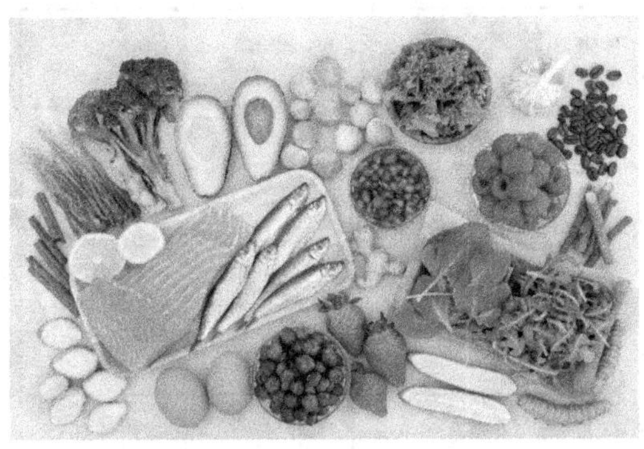

Fruits	Vegetables	Spices/Herbs	Superfoods/Other	Whole Grains
Berries	Bok Choy	Turmeric	Cocoa	Amaranth
Cherries	Zucchini	Rosemary	Dark Chocolate 70%	Barley
Avocado	Spinach	Ginger	Almonds, Cashews	Brown Rice
Citrus Fruits	Kale	Cinnamon	Pecans	Oats
Melons	Cucumber	Mint	Pine Nuts	Quinoa
Bananas	Collards	Cumin	Walnuts	Wild Rice
Apples	Brussel Sprouts	Black Pepper	Salmon	Millet
Pears	Potatoes	Clove	Mackerel	Brown Rice Pasta
Cherries	Sweet	Curry	Tuna	Wheat

	Potatoes			Berries
Grapes	Squash	Garlic	Sardines	Bulgar
Pomegranate	Peas	Mustard	Seeds: Chia, Flax	
Dried Fruits	Root Vegetables	Nutmeg	Hemp, pumpkin	
Mangos	Seaweed	Paprika	Beans/Legumes (see cooking instructions)	
Pineapples	Fermented Veggies	Basil	Greek Yogurt/Kefir	
Papayas	Mushrooms	Chives	Extra Virgin Olive Oil	
Peaches	Onion	Cilantro	Avocado Oil	
Cranberries	Garlic	Dill	Coconut Oil	
Dragon Fruit	Peppers	Sage	Walnut Oil	
Plantains	Cabbage	Oregano	Hemp Oil	
Kiwi	Beets	Thyme	Eggs	
Dates	Golden Beets	Tarragon	Chicken/Turkey	
Prunes	Leafy Greens	Parsley	Wild Game	
JackFruit	Artichoke	Cardamom		
Kumquat	Asparagus	Ginseng		

Lichee	Carrots	Green Tea		

Example List of Foods to Avoid from www.nutrition.va.gov:

Choose these foods LESS often. They can contribute to more inflammation.

Hydrogenated/ Trans Fat	Excess and Added Sugar	Food Additives	Sweeteners	Processed Meats
Check food labels for "partially hydrogenated oil" listed in the ingredients list. It may be found in: • Fried foods • High fat sauces • Creamy dressings • Baked goods • Crackers • Packaged snacks • Fast food • Peanut butter • Margarine • Shortening *Partially hydrogenated oils have been banned by the FDA and will be eliminated from food distribution by January 1, 2021*	**Sweet Beverages** • Sports drinks • Soda/pop • Energy drinks • Juice • Sweet coffee drinks **Sweets, desserts, and candy** **Added Sugar:** • Agave nectar • Beet sugar • Brown sugar • Confectioners' sugar (powdered sugar) • Corn syrup • Cane sugar • High fructose corn syrup (HFCS) • Honey • Maple syrup • Molasses • Organic, raw sugar 1 teaspoon sugar= 4 grams of sugar	**Additives** • Artificial flavors • Artificial colors • BHA • BHT • MSG • Nitrates/Nitrites • Polysorbate 80 • Added phosphates • Soy protein isolate **Examples of foods that contain these:** • Ready-to-eat meals (TV dinners) • Chips • Packaged cookies • Packaged crackers Start reading the ingredients label on any food you buy in a can, bag, box, or package. Look for these food additives!	**Artificial Sweeteners** (Avoid) • Acesulfame K (Ace K, Sweet One) • Aspartame (Equal, NutraSweet) • Saccharin (Sweet N' Low) • Sucralose (Splenda) **Sugar Alcohols** (Use with caution) • Erythritol • Maltitol • Mannitol • Sorbitol • Xylitol Natural Sweeteners (Use sparingly) • Monk fruit • Stevia	• Bacon • Bologna • Bratwurst • Corned beef • Deli meat • Ham • Pepperoni • Hot dogs • Salami • Sausage • Spam

Cooking Methods:

According to John Hopkins Medical, it is best to prepare your foods raw, steamed, baked or stir fried when trying to reduce inflammation. Grilling meats can produce compounds that are associated with cancer, however, if you grill low-fat fish or vegetables these same compounds are not produced, so these are good alternative foods to cook on the grill. Deep frying causes the food to be high in fat and can cause an inflammatory response. Rinse beans and legumes and, soak in water for 5 hours. Then boil in fresh water for 30 minutes. This will help them to be more easily digestible.

Portion Size: Easy Portioning

There are some easy tools you can use to help you understand and follow proper food portioning. These methods are not exact but represent a close visual of how you should be portioning your meals. I often do not measure with spoons and cups but use these two techniques to guide me. This saves time and dirty dishes! However, when you are completing your 1st cleanse and 28-day anti-inflammatory meal plan, I highly recommend that you measure! This will help you to understand what your portions should look like regularly.

Hand Portioning:

Tip of Index Finger= 1 Teaspoon (Use for measuring oils, butter and mayo, etc.)
Thumb= 1 Tablespoon (Use to measure salad dressing, nut butter, etc.)
Cupped Hand = 1 ounce (used for measuring snacks)
Palm of Hand= 3oz (You should eat 3 to 4 oz of meat per serving, so use to measure the meat proteins in your meals)
Fist= 1 Cup (use to measure fruit, rice, quinoa, oatmeal, etc.)

Plate Portioning: Plan Your Plate

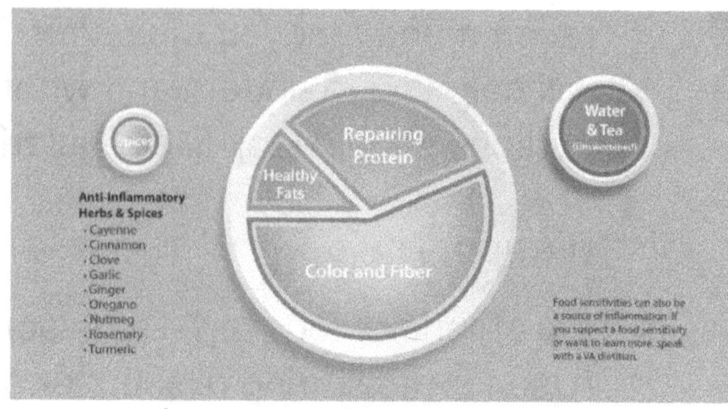

(www.nutrition.va.gov)

Tips for Eating Out

It is best if you try not to eat out for the first 30 days of the program…even waiting 2 weeks would be a huge gift to your body. We know the reality is that we often are on the go or want to enjoy a night out on the town with friends! And I will say…this is doable! We just must change how we approach the menu and our portion sizing! Here is how:

*Choose restaurants that can support your positive eating choices and stay away from fast food!

*Select foods that are not fried or cooked in a lot of oils, or kindly ask if they can reduce the number of oils they use. For example, my husband and I love veggie fajitas, and they can be a good choice when eating out, but unfortunately, they are often saturated in oil when delivered to the table. Now, when ordering, we politely ask if they can make it without the oil or greatly reduce the oil, and we always have a backup order in case it is not possible!

*Share a meal. This reduces the portion size to a reasonable amount and helps to reduce food waste. If sharing isn't an option, ask for a box at the beginning of the meal and split your portion before starting to eat. This eliminates the desire to clear your plate and the mindless picking of food after you are full.

*Look for a meal that is well balanced with a good lean protein and packed with anti-inflammatory veggies etc. An example might be a salmon with asparagus and rice or a steak with broccolini. Or perhaps...a veggie rice bowl. You can even order a hamburger without the bun and a salad as your side. Get creative and have fun!

*Order an iced tea or sparkling water in a fancy wine glass and skip the alcohol. Or order a really delicious glass of wine and savor every sip (you can replace your last snack of the day with a 6oz glass of red wine).

*Order berries and whipped cream for dessert or skip it all together. You know you have yummy options that you can eat when you get home.

*Consider meals with more nutrient density and less fats and sugars.

*Be present and in the moment and enjoy every joyful minute of your night out!

Some suggestions for fast food on the go:
- Starbucks protein plate
- MOD Pizza build your own pizza with a gluten free crust, red sauce, lots of veggies and only a sprinkle of cheese...don't forget the garlic and fresh basil!
- Simple sushi roll with rice, fish and avocado
- Panera salad and soup combo
- Thai Curry

*Build your Own Salad Bar...beware of the salad trap! Many salads contain very high caloric dressing and preserved meat. For example, Caesar salad can have over 1000 calories in one serving! Applebee's Cesar salad, for example, says it contains 970 calories. Instead, opt for a mixed green salad with veggies and a yummy vinaigrette. You can even top with a sprinkle of feta or parmesan.

*And...don't forget to keep drinking water! Water helps to bring nutrients to the cells, eliminate waste, protect our organs and joints and maintain body temperature! Choose water over other drink options when eating out on the go!

How to Survive the Weekends?!

The weekends can be challenging as we often have social events to attend and more time on our hands to revert back to our old eating habits. I know that I still struggle with this, and want to share a few suggestions on how to make the weekends successful and positive!

*Host events at your house, so you can control the food options.

*Enlist friends and ask them to prepare a weekend meal with you!

*Stay busy and active. If you are feeling like you just want to give up for the weekend, engage in something you enjoy or get outside and go for a walk or hike. If the weather is bad, you can go to the mall and do laps.

*When attending social gatherings, bring some of your healthy snacks to share. Make yummy appetizers to share that you can enjoy. You will be surprised how many people will ask for the recipes!

*Make mocktails with sparkling water, mint and lime. Then serve in a fancy glass or big chunky wine glass and add an orange or lime to the rim. I believe that a big part of our enjoyment of cocktail hour is the ritual of the glass! If you know me, you know that I LOVE A BIG CHUNKY WINE GLASS even if it is filled with iced tea or sparkling water!

*Meal prep for the following week!

*Enjoy yummy meals from the meal plan. Remember, I try to make all the dinners on the plan sharable, and there are some special yummy weekend family dinners!

*Note: If you are a person who really loves your glass of red wine, and feels it has a healthy effect, you can add in **one 6oz glass** of red wine to replace your last snack of the day. If you choose to do this, take note in your journal because several of my clients recognized that it causes them stomach upset and difficulty sleeping. This is because they have cut it out of their diet for at least two weeks and can be very inflammatory for some!

28-Day Anti-Inflammatory Meal Plan Recipes

Smoothie Recipes:

Blueberry Peach Smoothie

1 cup fresh blueberries
1 cup frozen peaches
1 cup almond milk
½ cup Greek yogurt or kefir
2 tablespoons hemp seed
Place all items in a blender and blend until smooth.
Note: This recipe will make two smoothies, so you can save one for later or share with someone you love!

Oatmeal Smoothie

¼ cup gluten free whole grain oats
1 frozen banana
½ cup unsweetened almond or coconut milk
1 tablespoon creamy peanut butter

½ teaspoon pure vanilla extract
½ teaspoon ground cinnamon
½ tablespoon pure grade maple
syrup
Handful of spinach or kale

- Blend and enjoy!

Pineapple Enzyme Smoothie

1 cup pineapple chunks
1 small banana
1 scoop vanilla protein powder
½ cup almond or coconut milk
1 handful spinach
Handful of ice

- Blend and Enjoy

Berry-Watermelon Smoothie

1 cup watermelon or melon of choice
¾ cup blueberries
2 tablespoons hemp seeds
Handful of spinach or kale
1 scoop of vanilla protein
Handful of ice

- Blend until smooth and serve

Fat Burning Pineapple Smoothie

½ cup nut milk of choice
¼ cup fresh squeezed orange juice
1 small frozen banana
Handful of greens
1 scoop clean vanilla protein
1 teaspoon cinnamon
- Blend until smooth and serve

Chai Vanilla Smoothie

½-¾ cup nut milk
Handful of spinach
Small amount of fresh ginger root (or you can used powdered ginger)
½ frozen banana
1 scoop clean vanilla protein powder
Chai Spice Mix: nutmeg, cardamom, black pepper, and cinnamon
1 tablespoon clean nut butter of choice
1 tablespoon hemp seed

- Blend until smooth and serve

Orange, Mango, Vanilla Smoothie

½ cup coconut water
Handful of greens (spinach or kale)
¼ -½ cup fresh squeezed orange juice
½ frozen banana
½ cup mango
Sprig of fresh basil
Sprig of fresh mint
Small drizzle of honey

- Blend until smooth and serve

Banana Chocolate Heaven Smoothie

1 cup nut milk of choice
Handful of spinach
½ frozen banana
1 scoop of cacao powder (about 1 ½ tablespoons)
¼ cup uncooked gluten free oats
1 teaspoon of honey
1 tablespoon peanut butter optional
(only ingredient in your peanut butter

should be peanuts and can contain salt)

- Blend until smooth and serve

Chocolate Dinner Smoothie

1 cup nut milk of choice
¼ cup water
Handful of spinach
½ frozen banana
1 scoop of cacao powder (about 1 ½ tablespoons)
¼ cup uncooked gluten free oats
1 teaspoon hemp seeds
1 tablespoon peanut butter
¼ avocado
1 teaspoon cinnamon
½ teaspoon honey
Small handful of ice

- Blend until smooth and serve

Note: I eat the avocado on the side, but if you put it into a smoothie, you have a thick and creamy shake.

Mixed Berry Bliss Smoothie

¾ cup coconut water or coconut milk
½ cup kefir
½ cup mixed berries of choice
½ banana
Handful of greens (spinach or kale)
½ scoop of clean vanilla protein
1 tablespoon hemp or chia seeds
  - Blend until smooth and serve

Inflammation Buster Pina Colada Smoothie

1 cup coconut water
½ cup fresh pineapple
Handful of greens (spinach or kale)
¼ cup of cucumber
Drizzle of honey
½ teaspoon of coconut oi
2 tablespoons fresh coconut
  - Blend until smooth and serve

Strawberry Vanilla Smoothie

1 cup water or coconut water
Handful of greens

1 cup strawberries
1 small frozen banana (if using an unfrozen banana add ¼ cup ice)
1 scoop clean vanilla powder

- Blend until smooth and serve

Melon Ginger Smoothie

¾ cup water or coconut water
¾ cup watermelon or cantaloupe
¾ cup blueberries
2 tablespoons fresh ginger
Handful of greens
1 scoop clean vanilla protein powder
1 tablespoon hemp seeds
¼ cup ice
- Blend until smooth and serve

Refreshing Turmeric Smoothie

1 cup nut milk of choice
1 1/12 cups of pineapple chunks
1 banana
Handful of greens

1 tablespoon of fresh turmeric or you can replace with ground turmeric 1 ½ tsp
1 1/2 teaspoon of fresh ginger or can replace with ½ teaspoon of ground ginger
Mint sprigs

- Blend until smooth and serve

Berry Basil Smoothie

1 cup coconut water
1 handful of greens
1 cup of fresh strawberries
½ cup of frozen berries of choice
1 tablespoon lemon juice
¼ cup basil (fresh)
Mint sprigs
½ teaspoon fresh local honey

- Blend until smooth and serve

Green Smoothie

½ cup nut milk of choice
¼ cup water
1 small green pear chopped

Large handful of greens
¼ cup cucumber
1 ½ teaspoon of fresh ginger or can replace with ½ teaspoon of ground ginger
1 teaspoon hemp seeds
1 teaspoon fresh local honey
- Blend until smooth and serve

Fall Spice Smoothie (Delicious Any Time of Year!)

¾ cup nut milk
¼ cup ice
Handful of greens
1 frozen banana
½ cup pumpkin puree 100% puree organic
¾ cup apple cut into small pieces
½ tablespoon maple syrup
1 1/2 teaspoon of fresh ginger or can replace with ½ teaspoon of ground ginger
½ teaspoon cinnamon
Dash of nutmeg
Dash of clove

1 tsp vanilla

- Blend until smooth and serve

Strawberry Peach Smoothie

1 cup frozen strawberry
1 cup frozen peaches
1 cup almond milk
½ cup greek yogurt or kefir
¼ cup frozen dark cherries
2 pitted dates
2 tablespoons hemp seed
Place all items in a blender and blend until smooth.
Note: This recipe will make two smoothies, so you can save one for later or share with someone you love!

Soup Recipes:

Kabocha Thai Soup

1 large kabocha squash (cut into quarters and remove the seeds) You

can also use butternut or acorn squash or in a hurry substitute 2 cans of pumpkin.

¼ cup thinly sliced ginger
3 cloves garlic, minced
1 yellow onion, chopped
4 cups of chicken bone broth or veggie stock
1 can coconut milk full fat
2 tablespoons curry paste-I use red or yellow
Sprinkle of sea salt and pepper
2 limes cut into thirds
Basil fresh chopped for topping
Red chili slices for topping if desired

- Preheat oven to 350
- Place squash on a large roasting pan with the cut side up
- Divide ginger slices and garlic between each cavity and sprinkle a little water
- Arrange the onions around the squash

- Pour 2 cups of broth into roasting pan and discover with foil
- Bake for one hour and a half until squash is completely cooked
- While waiting for veggies to cook in the oven , take out a soup pan and saute the curry paste in 2 teaspoons of olive oil. Let cool and wait to add remaining ingredients
- Transfer the vegetables (make sure to do it carefully because they are hot!) to a soup pan
- Scoop out the squash into the soup pan
- Add remaining broth, coconut milk, salt and pepper and bring to a boil
- Reduce to medium heat and simmer for 10 minutes
- Using an immersion blender puree until creamy

- Top with lime, basil and optional peppers

Cold Cantaloupe Soup

1 Large cantaloupe
½ cup fresh squeezed orange juice
¼ cup honey
1 cup greek yogurt or plain kefir
1 tablespoon apple cider vinegar
Basil and mint sprigs

- Cut melon and remove all seeds
- Cut melon into cubes and place in bowl
- Add the orange juice, yogurt , honey, vinegar
- Use immersion blender and blend until smooth
- Chill in refrigerator
- Serve in a cute bowl or stemless wine glass

Breakfast Recipes:

Ezekiel Raisin French Toast

2 eggs
¼ cup almond milk
½ teaspoon vanilla extract
4 pieces of Ezekiel Raisin Bread
4 tablespoons pure grade maple syrup
4 pieces of uncured bacon

- Beat together eggs, almond milk and vanilla extract
- Dip each piece of raisin bread into egg mixture and coat
- Prepare bacon
- Heat pan to medium heat and add 1 tsp olive oil to pan
- Place bread in pan and cook on both sides
- Top with maple syrup and serve with 2 pieces of toast and 2 pieces of bacon

Note: This makes 2 servings

Easy Breakfast Burrito

¼ cup peppers
½ cup zucchini
3 tablespoons chopped onions
3 eggs
¼ cup black beans or beans of choice
2 tablespoons grated mozzarella
2 tablespoons salsa
Gluten free tortilla

- Saute peppers, zucchini and onions in 1 tablespoon avocado oil
- Add in eggs and scramble
- Add in the beans and spoon mixture over gluten free tortilla
- Top with mozzarella and salsa

Maple Pecan Quinoa

¼ c quinoa cooked
½ c almond or coconut milk
½ tsp vanilla
2 tablespoon chopped pecans
½ cup berries of choice

- Pre-cook quinoa and measure out ¼ cup to warm up
- Top with ingredients
- Add one tablespoon of honey or maple syrup (I like maple syrup with this one!)

Oatmeal Banana Pancakes

2 tablespoons avocado oil
2 egg whites or 1 large egg
1 scoop clean vanilla protein
4 tablespoons slow cooked gluten free oats
Half of a large banana mashed
2 tablespoons water
1/2 teaspoon pure vanilla extract (optional)
1 teaspoon cinnamon

- Heat up avocado oil in pan on medium heat
- Mix together all remaining ingredients by hand.
- Spoon in pancake mixture to form a pancake

- Cook until brown and flip…cook opposite side until brown
- Serve with 1 teaspoon of grassfed butter and 2 tablespoons pure grade maple syrup.

2 Egg Scramble

2 eggs scrambled
¼ cup spinach
2 tablespoons chopped sweet yellow onion
¼ cup mushrooms
1 tablespoon avocado oil
2 tablespoons clean salsa
¼ avocado

- Place spinach, onions, and mushrooms in a pan and saute in avocado oil for two minutes.
- Add in scrambled eggs and cook.

- Toss in spinach and cook for an additional minute.
- Top with salsa and avocado and serve!

Avocado Toast

1 slice of Eziekel or Fresh Fermented Sourdough
½ avocado
1 finely chopped clove of garlic
sea salt and pepper to taste
½ teaspoon lemon juice
1 egg either fried or sliced hard boiled
Garlic powder to taste preference

- Toast bread
- Cut and pit avocado
- While the bread is toasting…place all other ingredients in a bowl and mash together with a fork.
- Spread on toast
- Top with Egg and Enjoy!

Spinach Egg Scramble with Berries

1 teaspoon grass fed or amish butter
1 ½ cups baby spinach
2 large eggs slightly beaten
Pinch of salt and pepper
1 slice of fresh sourdough or ezekiel bread
½ cup fresh berries of choice

- Place butter in pan over medium heat
- Scramble eggs, add spinach, and add salt and pepper
- Serve the eggs and spinach over toast with the ½ cup berries

Avocado and Spinach Omelet

2 large eggs
1 teaspoon almond milk
2 tablespoons avocado oil (divided)
1 cup chopped spinach fresh or frozen
2 tablespoons onion

1 tablespoon lime juice
1 tablespoon chopped fresh cilantro
1 teaspoon papitas
Pinch of crushed red pepper
Pinch of salt
Pinch of pepper
1 tablespoon shaved parmesan
½ avocado sliced

- Beat eggs with almond milk and salt in small bowl
- Heat 1 teaspoon oil in a small nonstick skillet over medium heat
- Pour in egg mixture to skillet
- Cook until center is set and still a little runny in the middle
- Flip over and cook until firm…about 30 seconds
- Transfer to plate
- Place the remaining teaspoon of oil into the skillet and toss in kale, lime juice, cilantro, seeds, red pepper and a pinch of

salt/pepper until kale begins to wilt and crisp
- Remove from pan and place atop the eggs
- Sprinkle with parmesan
- Add avocado and serve! Delicious!

Apple, Raisin Oatmeal

½ cup oatmeal

½ chopped apple

¼ cup raisins

1 teaspoon cinnamon

1 teaspoon pure grade A maple syrup

½ teaspoon avocado oil

- Place avocado oil in pot and heat on low-medium heat

- Place apples and cinnamon in the pot and saute for 1 minute in oil
- Add in oatmeal and water to cooking specifications
- Spoon in th maple syrup and raisin and mix
- Cook until done…Eat! YUM!

2 Eggs, Bacon and Sourdough Toast

2 eggs prepared to your liking in 1 tablespoon avocado oil
2 slices of bacon
1 piece of sourdough toast with ½ teaspoon of butter or 1 teaspoon of nut butter
Prepare and enjoy!

Lunch/Dinner Recipes:

Note: Many of the dinner item recipes are portioned to prepare for family meals, if you only need 1 portion, you can use as leftovers or freeze. Make sure to always adhere to propper portion sizing!

Anti-Inflammatory Lasagna

- Prepare brown rice noodles as specified on package
- Saute veggies of choice in pan with garlic and oil
- Cook ground turkey and season with oregano, basil, garlic powder etc to taste
- Spray a rectangle glass baking dish with cooking spray
- Layer the ingredients starting with noodles, ground turkey, veggies, sauce and continue building the layers to cover and fill baking dish
- Sprinkle with the mozzarella and parm
- Bake at 375 degrees for 35-45 minutes
- Top with fresh basil (can use basil spice if no fresh basil available)

- You can add a dollop of greek yogurt if you like the creamy addition to your lasagne!
- Serve with a salad and homemade dressing

Note: I love italian spices so I always add extra and even throw in some red pepper flakes

Thai Chicken Lettuce Wraps

1 tablespoon full fat greek yogurt
1 tablespoon fresh or spice basil
1 tsp minced garlic
1 teaspoon lime juiceBrown Rice Lasagna Noodles
1 jar of organic, no sugar added spaghetti sauce
1 tablespoon avocado oil
3 cloves garlic, minced
1 pound ground turkey
2 cups Mixed veggies of choice sauteed
½ cup mozzarella ¼ cup parmesan
Fresh Basil to top

½ cup sliced chicken
¼ cup chopped red onions
½ cup chopped mushrooms
½ cup cooked brown rice
2 Butter Lettuce Leaves

- Mix together greek yogurt, basil, garlic, lime juice in a medium bowl
- Add chicken, red onions, mushrooms to mixture
- Split half cup of brown rice in two and spoon over the two lettuce leaves
- Top with chicken mixture and enjoy!

Tip: Double this recipe and eat for two lunches in a row to make prepping easier!

Veggie Enchiladas

2 sweet potatoes cooked, peeled and mashed
1 can sweet corn
1 can black beans
½ yellow onion sliced

3 cloves garlic, diced
1 zucchini chopped in squares
1 bunch of broccoli or cauliflower
chopped and steamed
1 tsp ground cumin
5 to six ounces of ground spinach
8 whole wheat or clean corn tortillas
Homemade enchilada sauce or 1 can
red enchilada and one can clean
ingredient cream of chicken soup
1/4 cup grated mozzarella or cotija
cheese to top for flavoring before
baking
Handful of cilantro to top

- Preheat oven to 400 degrees
- Bake sweet potatoes ahead
- Lightly grease a 9 by 13 inch pan with olive oil or cooking spray
- In large skillet over medium heat warm olive oil and add onions, garlic, zucchini and salt and cook stirring often for about 5 minutes

- Add in broccoli, corn, salt and cumin until warm…then add the spinach and cook for additional 2 minutes
- Transfer to a large mixing bowl and blend in sweet potatoes- this is your filling
- Open the cans and pour the enchilada sauce and cream of chicken soup into a large skillet and heat until both blend together smoothly to make the sauce and then turn off the burner.-this is your sauce

Assemble the enchiladas

- Pour ¼ cup of the enchilada sauce into the prepared pan and move from side to side until evenly coated
- Dip each tortilla into the sauce (coating both sides)
- Place a large amount of filling in the middle and roll

- Place each rolled tortilla in the prepared pan with seam side down side by side
- Drizzle the remaining sauce
- Sprinkle with cheese on top and bake for about 20 minutes on middle rack

Note: You can serve with a dollop of greek yogurt to substitute sour cream.

Quinoa Acorn Squash (p43 sp ed ce anti-inflammatory)

Baked Sweet Potato and Salad

2 large sweet potatoes washed and prepped (you will prepare both and save one)
1 ½ tablespoon olive oil or avocado oil
1 small garlic clove crushed
½ cup of slivered almonds or pine nuts
1 cup of kale
¼ cup hummus
Salad per lunch:

½ cup mixed green or salad veggies of choice
2 tablespoons lemon juice mixed with ½ teaspoon of oil and spices of choice

- Place a piece of foil over baking sheet
- Preheat oven to 425 degrees
- Use fork to puncture holes
- Set on baking sheet and bake for 40 to 50 minutes until fully cooked
- On an additional baking sheet, spread out the kale and almonds, sprinkle with sea salt, garlic
- Drizzle the olive oil evenly over the kale and almonds and bake for 3-5 minutes
- Slice baked potato in half and top with kale and almonds
- Prepare salad
- Plate with topped potato and salad and enjoy-Reserve the

second potato and half of the kale/almond mixture for another lunch or dinner this week!

Note: If you are in a hurry,you can just top the sweet potato with the almonds and drizzle a ½ teaspoon of maple syrup.

Avocado Toast

1 slice of Eziekel or Fresh Fermented Sourdough
½ avocado
1 finely chopped clove of garlic
sea salt and pepper to taste
½ teaspoon lemon juice
1 egg either fried or sliced hard boiled
Garlic powder to taste preference

- Toast bread
- Cut and pit avocado
- While bread is toasting…place all other ingredients in a bowl and mash together with fork.
- Spread on toast
- Top with Egg and Enjoy!

Veggie Beet Hummus Wrap

2 tablespoons Hummus (see hummus recipe in snack area of 28 day meal plan)
1 6 inch Sprouted Grain or Gluten Free Tortilla
½ cup shredded golden beets
¼ cup chopped cucumber
Sprinkle of chopped red onion
¼ cup packed greens (spinach, arugula, kale or spring mix)
2 tablespoons clean fresh feta
1 tablespoon oregano
1 tablespoon basil or chopped fresh basil

- Prepare tortilla with hummus spread
- Top evenly with all other ingredients.
- Roll tightly like a burrito
- Wrap in foil or parchment and place in refrigerator until served

These are great on the go! Just place the wrapped wrap in a plastic baggy and take with you! You can do any variation of vegetables with this wrap.

Unbelievable Carrot Hot Dog:

8 Carrots Peeled (select carrots that are hot dog size)

Prepare the Marinade by mixing the following ingredients in a bowl:

¼ c Coconut Aminos
¼c apple Cider vinegar with mother
¼ c mustard of choice
2 Tbs Maple Syrup
3 tsp garlic minced
1 tsp garlic powder
½ tsp onion powder
1 Tbs Liquid Smoke

- Trim and peel carrots and place in boiling water for about 10 minutes (until tender)
- Drain the carrots with cold water and make sure they are cool
- Add the mixed marinade and the carrots to a ziplock bag and seal
- Place in the refrigerator
- Let marinate for at least 8 hours (longer if possible)
- Grill or Air Fry the carrots until warm throughout and have some grill marks
- Place the carrot dog on a gluten free or sourdough hotdog bun
- Top with your favorite hotdog garnished

Healthy Portuguese Green Soup:

2 Tbl avocado oil

1 Large Yellow Onion
4 cloves of garlic sliced
6 Medium Yukon Gold potatoes,
peeled and chopped into 4ths
2-3 large carrots peeled and chopped
in thirds
4 cups vegetable broth
½ pound of spinach or kale
Veggies of choice for the soup
(chopped for soup)
Fresh grass fed sausage or Aidells
Chicken Apple Sausage (omit if
making vegetarian/Vegan)
Sea salt, pepper, oregano, garlic
powder and basil to taste

1. Boil the potatoes and carrots
   until tender and let cool down
   for 5 minutes
2. Saute the garlic and onion in
   the avocado and let cool
3. Place the potatoes, carrots,
   onion, garlic and some of the
   water from the boiling pot into a
   blender or use an emulsifier to
   blend together until creamy.

4. Saute the spinach in water and lightly saute any additional vegetables from the anti-inflammatory list that you wish to add to the soup.
5. Cook the sausage (if using in recipe)
6. Add blended base, 4 cups of vegetable broth, sausage and veggies to warm.
7. Add spices and let simmer for 3-5 minutes
8. Serve and Enjoy!
9. Note: You can use the base (steps 1-3 and veggie broth) to make any soup mixture! You can even add shrimp! Yum!

Bacon and Avocado Sandwich with Green Salad

Sandwich:

1 slice fresh sourdough bread
3-4 slices of uncured cooked bacon
½ avocado

Sprinkle of garlic powder
2 tablespoons of garlic or spicy
avocado hummus
Lettuce of choice to top sandwich

- Toast the piece of sourdough
- Spread humus evenly over slice
  of bread
- Mash avocado and add a
  sprinkle of garlic powder
- Spread Avocado over bread
- Top with bacon and lettuce
- I eat this as an open face
  sandwich, but you can also
  make it into a half sandwich!

Small Green Salad:

½ cup of mixed greens or spinach
½ cup of veggies of choice to add to
salad
2 tablespoons sliced almonds

- Mix lettuce and veggies
  together and top with fresh
  lemon juice and olive oil.

Southwest Chicken Wrap

1 Large Romaine Leaf

1/2 c. Shredded Lettuce

1/3 c. Black Beans

¼ cup sweet corn

1/2 c. chicken sliced into small pieces

3 tablespoons chopped red onions

1 tbsp. Salsa

Sprinkle of Cilantro

Sprinkle of lime juice

Sprinkle of Cotija Cheese (very small amount…just to give flavoring)

Sprinkle of oregano, salt, pepper, garlic pepper and cayenne

- Mix together in a bowl
- Spoon into lettuce leaves and enjoy!

Taco Tuesday

1 pound meat of choice: chicken, grass fed ground beef or wild caught with fish

1 tablespoon avocado oil

6 inch gluten free or ezekiel tortillas (or I love the cauliflower tortillas in frozen section)

For seasoning:

1 tablespoon chili powder

1 teaspoon oregano

1 teaspoon onion powder

1 teaspoon garlic powder

1 teaspoon paprika

½ teaspoon cumin

For topping:

½ onion diced

¼ -½ head of lettuce chopped or bag of broccoli coleslaw

1 small can sliced olives

Shredded feta, mozzarella or parmesan (just to sprinkle with taste) approx 2 tablespoon serving

1 avocado cubed

Dollop of greek yogurt per taco

For Beans:
1 can pinto beans
4 cloves of garlic finely chopped
2 slices of cooked uncured bacon
with grease reserved for sauteing the
garlic
For rice:
2 cups cooked brown rice
⅓ cup clean salsa

- Prepare seasoning by mixing together all ingredients for seasoning in a jar.
- Prepare meat of choice and place in a pan with olive oil. Spoon in 2-3 tablespoons of seasoning. You can season to taste after the meat is cooked if you want to add more flavor. Cook meat completely.
- Cook two pieces of uncured bacon and reserve the grease
- Cook brown rice in the rice cooker while preparing taco beans and filling.

- In a separate pot place the reserved bacon grease and 4 garlic cloves finely chopped. And cook for two minutes. Then add pinto beans and warm. Break in the bacon bits and mash the beans with a masher. Delicious and healthy refried beans!
- Prepare taco toppings for build your own taco bar.
- When rice is completely cooked…spoon in the salsa and mix. Easy Spanish rice.
- Place spoons in the rice and beans and Taco Tuesday is ready to begin!

Note: Pay attention to your portioning here! We tend to get excited and forget to adhere to the correct portion sizes. I like to eat mine over the lettuce and skip the tortilla or make lettuce wraps for myself and serve the family tortillas. So a palm of hand for meat (3-4 oz), fist of rice (1 cup) or less and ½ fist (½ cup of beans) will make a good plate portion! The lettuce and veggies are unlimited and the cheese and greek yogurt should be approximately 2 Thumbs (2 tablespoons max).

Lemongrass and Ginger Chicken

8 large chicken thighs
4 garlic cloves chopped
2 tablespoons fish sauce
1 tablespoon honey
1 cup water
3 sticks of lemongrass finely chopped
3 tablespoons, fresh, ginger root, peeled and chopped
2 tablespoons of avocado oil
2 limes (1 for juicing and one to slice and serve with meal)
2 tbsp, coriander chopped.
1 and 1/2 cups, Jasmine rice uncooked.

- Mix honey and fish sauce in large bowl and add chicken
- Coat the chicken completely cover and marinate in fridge for 30 minutes
- Prepare and cook 1 ½ cups of jasmine rice in rice cooker
- Blend lemongrass, ginger and chopped garlic in a food processor.
- Heat oil in large pan
- add chicken (reserving marinade to add later) and brown well
- Add lemon grass mixture
- Cook until fragrant
- Add marinade and 1 cup water- stir well and cover
- Simmer over low heat for 30 to 35 minutes
- Remove from heat and add lemon juice and coriander…you can taste and adjust to your liking

- Serve with Jasmine rice and a small slices of lime

Note: I also like to add fresh chopped basil, mint and thai basil! Yummy!

Healthy Pad Thai

½ to ¾ package of Pad Thai Rice Noodles (I get the fresh ones at the Asian Market)

3 tablespoons avocado oil

1 lb boneless and skinless chicken breasts chopped (optional) Add more veggies if you do not use the chicken.

½ cup of bell peppers sliced (I prefer red for this recipe)

2 cup carrots sliced into thin pieces

1/2 cup chopped yellow onion

3 tablespoon garlic minced

½ bag of frozen peas

½ cup zucchini

2 eggs

For the sauce:

3 tablespoons peanut butter (all natural with only peanuts)

3 tablespoons pure grade maple syrup or honey

3 tablespoons lime juice

2+ tablespoons rice wine vinegar

1 tablespoon fish sauce

½ tablespoon sriracha

¼-½ cup coconut aminos (you can use low sodium soy as substitute.)

Toppings:

- red pepper flakes or chile sauce (optional)
- lime wedges
- chopped cilantro
- chopped mint
- chopped thai basil
- chopped basil
- bean sprouts
- ⅓ cup chopped peanuts or cashews
-

1. Chop vegetables to prepare for cooking.
2. Chop chicken into small squares and saute in a large pan over medium heat using

the avocado oil. Make sure that chicken is fully cooked.

3. At the same time boil water and prepare the thai noodles by following directions on the package.

4. Remove chicken from the saute pan when cooked, but leave the oil in the pan. Add the peppers, carrots, garlic and onion to the oil and saute for about 4-6 minutes.

5. Scoot the veggies to one side of the pan and crack the two egg into the pan and scramble. This will take about two minutes.

6. Add the noodles and sauce mixture to the pan and fold in

the noodles with the veggie mixture, sauce and noodles.

7. Add the frozen peas and cook for about 2 minutes, stirring regularly.

8. Toss in the chicken to warm.

9. Garnish with the toppings as preferred! The toppings make the dish so be generous!

Note: You can always make a little extra sauce and add if you like your noodles more saucy! :) ENJOY!

Chicken Pesto Avocado Boats

- 1 pound shredded cooked chicken
- ½ cup cranberries
- ¼ cup pine nuts

Pesto:

- 2 cups fresh basil leaves

- ½ cup pine nuts
- 1 tablespoon lemon juice
- 3 small garlic cloves
- ¼ cup extra virgin olive oil
- ¼ teaspoon sea salt
- ¼ cup parmesan cheese
- Ground black pepper

Blend all pesto ingredients together in a food processor or blender.

1. Halve and pit the avocados. Spoon out the avocado flesh from the skin, but leave a ¼ in the rim of the flesh.
2. Blend the basil, garlic, parm and olive oil in food processor to make pesto.
3. Fold the avocado flesh into the cooked chicken and stir.
4. Add the pesto, cranberries and pine nuts to the mixture.

5. Spoon into the avocado skins.

Serve and enjoy!

Mango Quinoa

1 cup spinach or kale
1 cup quinoa pre-cooked
½ cup yellow onion
½ cup Mango
½ cup coconut milk
¼ cup chopped almond
2 teaspoons avocado oil or coconut oil

- Sutee onions in oil for two minutes
- Add in quinoa, coconut milk and spinach and cook until spinach begins to wilt
- Remove from pan and place on plate.
- Top with mangos and chopped almonds and enjoy!

White Bean Salad

2 cups mixed salad greens
¾ cups chopped vegetables of choice
⅓ can of white beans rinsed and drained
½ avocado sliced
2 tablespoons feta cheese

Dressing:
1 tablespoon balsamic vinegar
½ tablespoon apple cider vinegar
2 tablespoons extra virgin olive oil
½ lemon juiced
1 clove garlic minced
Salt and pepper to taste

- Prepare dressing by shaking in a small glass jar
- Mix together all salad ingredients and toss with dressing. Enjoy!

Build Your Own Pizzas

For the crust: You can select gluten free tortillas such as sprouted or cauliflower, select a clean ingredient gluten free mix or make your own cauliflower or gluten free crust! Pizza should be the size of a 6 inch tortilla fajita size tortilla.

For the sauce (this is per tortilla portion, so make sure to make enough for each pizza you are preparing!):
2 tablespoons plain full fat greek yogurt
Teaspoon of basil
Teaspoon of oregano
1 clove chopped garlic
½ teaspoon of garlic powder (if you like garlic!)

For the toppings:
3 oz of cooked chicken per tortilla pizza

½ cup artichoke hearts per tortilla pizza
¼ of small red onion chopped
⅛ cu olives chopped per tortilla pizza
⅛ cup fetta or mozzarella cheese per tortilla pizza

- Place tortilla on parchment paper or pizza stone and pre-back for about 3 minutes
- Mix greek yogurt, spices and garlic together and spread even layer onto tortilla
- Top with toppings and cheese
- Bake at 375 degrees for about 8 minutes
- Pizza should be baked and crispy. Yum!

Note: You can substitute a clean red sauce and other vegetables for toppings. When making with your family you can prepare toppings to their tastes as well, so you can enjoy a family meal!

Taco Lettuce Wraps

1 lb 95% lean ground turkey or grass fed ground beef
3 cloves garlic
¾ cup chopped yellow onions
1 tablespoon olive oil
1 tablespoon chili powder
1 teaspoon ground cumin
½ teaspoon paprika
1 teaspoon oregano
½ cup tomato sauce
½ cup low sodium chicken bone broth
Salt and pepper
1 head butter leaf lettuce or hearts of romaine separated
1 diced avocado
¼ cup chopped cilantro
Grated cotija cheese just for spinning in the taste…no more than one tablespoon per wrap
Greek yogurt for topping in place of sour cream

- Heat olive oil and sauté onions

- Add meat and spices to the pan and cook about 5 minutes
- Add tomato sauce and broth and reduce heat to simmer for about 5 minutes until sauce has reduced down in the pan.
- Spoon meat mixture into lettuce wraps and top with avocado, cilantro, greek yogurt and a sprinkle of cheese. Make sure to adhere to portion sizing…typically around 3 wraps. Enjoy!

Anti-Inflammatory Chicken Piccata Casserole Recipe

2 tablespoons avocado oil
1 pound boneless, skinless chicken thighs cut into ½ inch pieces
2 tablespoons unsalted butter
1 lemon cut into slices
½ lemon juiced
3 teaspoons minced garlic
½ teaspoon salt divided
¼ teaspoon ground pepper

⅓ cup dry white wine

1 ½ cups chicken bone broth

2 tablespoons greek yogurt

8 cups chopped and steamed kale

1 cup whole wheat or gluten free orzo

2 tablespoons drained and chopped capers

1 tablespoon flat-leaf parsley

- Preheat oven to 400 degrees
- Heat oil in large skillet over medium heat
- Place chicken in large bowl and toss with ¼ teaspoon salt and ¼ teaspoon pepper.
- Add the chicken to the heated pan
- Cook until golden brown on each side
- Remove chicken and set aside… then place butter lemon juice and lemon slices in pan and cook for about 1 minute
- Set aside lemon mixture with the chicken

- Add orzo and garlic to the pan and cook stirring often until orzo is lightly browned (about 2-3 minutes)
- Add the wine and cook stirring constantly until mostly absorbed …about 1 minute
- Add broth, kale, capers and the remaining salt.
- Bring to a boil over high heat and return chicken and lemon mixture to the pan.
- Transfer mixture into an oven safe baking dish
- Bake until orzo is tender and the chicken is fully cooked. Approximately 10 minutes at 400 degrees.
- Sprinkle parsley and serve!

Chicken Salad-Salad

Dressing:

2 tablespoons extra virgin olive oil
1 lemon juiced

½ tablespoon fresh turmeric

1 teaspoon dijon or yellow mustard

½ teaspoon pepper

1 tablespoon local honey

2 cloves garlic

Chicken Salad:

3-4 oz of chicken breast

½ apple sliced

2 tablespoons chopped nuts of choice

3 tablespoons red onion

½ avocado sliced

1 cup of mixed greens

- Mix salad dressing ingredients
- Place mixed greens on plate and top with chicken, apple slices, onion, nuts and avocado
- Toss salad with dressing and enjoy!

Steak Night Dinner

4 ounces of grass fed steak of choice per person

1 large sweet potato per person

½ tablespoon grass fed butter per potato

Roasted Broccoli 1 cup per person

- Prepare steak to you liking
- Preheat oven to 375 degrees
- Bake sweet potato in oven at 375 until fully cooked and soft and top with butter
- Increase oven heat to 400 degrees
- Line baking sheet with parchment paper
- Toss broccoli florets with 1 tablespoon olive oil, salt, pepper and oregano and place on baking sheet
- Roast broccoli for 15 to 20 minutes or until browned.
- Serve the steak, potato and broccoli and enjoy! Happy SUNDAY!

Note: If you prefer not to eat meat on Sunday, you can replace the steak with a 4 ounces of flounder. Season and add lemon juice and bake at 375 degrees until flounder flakes easily with a fork, about 25 minutes.

Veggie Hummus Wrap

1 Lettuce Wrap Romaine (or 2 Butterleaf)
¼ cup hummus
Baby greens
¼ cup chopped cucumbers
½ cup quinoa or wild rice
½ bell pepper sliced
½ carrot chopped

- Mix together the ingredients and fill lettuce wrap. If you have extra filling it is ok to use additional pieces of lettuce.

Shrimp Thai Dinner

1 lb shrimp
1 pepper sliced (I like yellow or orange)
½ cup fresh basil or thai basil
¼ cup mint

1 lime wedged
1 tablespoon coconut oil
1 tablespoon ginger
1 cup brown rice uncooked-add 2
cups water and cook in rice cooker
prior to starting meal
Sauce:
2 tablespoons Liquid Coconut Aminos
11/2 cup pure grade A maple syrup
2 tablespoons lime juice
2 teaspoons sriracha

- Mix sauce ingredients in small
  bowl and set aside
- Pre-cook the brown rice
- Melt oil and saute ginger for
  approx 1 minute
- Add shrimp and cook for about
  3 minutes, add peppers and
  cook for about one minute
- Add sauce and cook on med-
  high for 1 minute
- Spoon shrimp mixture over the
  rice and top with basil and mint
  and a couple lime wedges

Delicious Lemon Pasta

½ cup Brown Rice Pasta or Fresh
Semolina Flour Pasta
3 oz cooked chicken, sliced and
cubed
4 tsp lemon juice
1 tsp olive oil (split)
½ cup chopped basil
3 cloves garlic minced
½ cup mushrooms
½ sweet yellow onion
Sprinkle of parmesan

- Saute garlic, onion until transparent
- Add mushrooms and chicken saute util chicken browned and cooked
- Prepare pasta
- Mix in additional ingredients and top with basil and a sprinkle of parm

Zoodle Shrimp Dinner

3 tablespoons unsalted grass fed or amish butter
3 tablespoons extra virgin olive oil
¼ cup shallot finely chopped
1 tablespoon white wine
2 tablespoons chicken or veggie broth
3 cloves of garlic finely minced
1 pound large shrimp peeled
6 cups zoodles or spaghetti squash (zoodles are zucchini noodles)
4 tablespoons grated parmesan cheese divided
2 tablespoons flat leaf parsley
4 tablespoons fresh basil
2 tablespoons oregano
2 tablespoons basil spice
2 tablespoons garlic powder
½ teaspoon pepper
½ teaspoon sea salt

- Heat butter and 1 tablespoon oil over medium heat

- Add shallots and garlic until fragrant…about 3 minutes
- Add wine and stock and cook until reduced
- Add shrimp, pepper and salt and cook until shrimp is thoroughly cooked-about 3 minutes
- Transfer shrimp to a plate but keep the sauce in skillet
- Add the remaining oil with zucchini noodles
- Return shrimp to skillet
- Cook stirring constantly until mixture is heated
- Add parmesan, parsley and basil and serve immediately

Easy Farro Bowl

1 cup Farro prepared or Quinoa
1 10 oz bag of mediterranean style salad kit (not using the package dressing)
8 oz of rotisserie chicken or home prepared chicken cubed

2 tablespoons sliced almonds
Dressing
½ lemon juiced
2 tablespoons balsamic
1 teaspoon local honey
Garlic powder to taste
Pepper to taste

- Prepare Farro according to package directions (I prepare this ahead of time when food prepping)
- Prepare dressing by mixing ingredients
- Toss ½ a bag of the mediterranean salad mix, 4 0z of chicken, and ½ of dressing into a bowl and top with 1 tablespoon almonds
- Save and store the other half of the ingredients for tomorrow's lunch!

Glazed Miso Salmon with Blanched Asparagus

1 tablespoon miso paste
1 tablespoon lime juice and sliced wedges
2 teaspoons coconut aminos
2 cloves garlic minced
1 teaspoon ground pepper
2 teaspoons honey
4 5 oz pieces of wild caught skin on salmon
¼ cup thinly sliced green onions
1 bunch of asperagus

- Preheat oven to broil and place the rack about 7 inches from heat source. I use my airfry setting on my oven.
- Line a rimmed backing pan with foil and lightly coat the foil with avocado oil cooking spray
- Whisk together lime juice, coconut aminos, honey, garlic and pepper in a small bowl

- Spread the miso mix over the 4 pieces of salmon evenly coating each piece
- Broil or air fry the filets of salmon until they easily flake-5-7 minutes
- While the salmon is cooking trim the asparagus and blanch in boiling water for about 1-2 minutes until cooked but still crisp-sprinkle with sea salt
- Plate the salmon and asparagus and sprinkle with green onions and serve with lime wedges

Lettuce Wrap Burgers with Sweet Potato Wedges and Salad

4 oz of grass fed ground beef plus additional beef for family
Toppings of choice for burgers
3-4 medium sweet potatoes
1 tablespoon avocado oil
Sprinkle of salt pepper and oregano

Romaine lettuce leafs for serving
4 cups mixed green salad
Prepared homemade dressing of
choice

- Form grassfed beef into 4 oz
  burgers
- Cut and prepare all toppings
  burger bar style
- Boil the sweet potatoes for 2
  minutes and remove from water
  and let cool down for a couple
  of minutes and then cut into
  wedges
- Mix the avocado oil into the
  potato wedges and place on a
  foil covered cooking sheet
- Sprinkle with salt, pepper and
  oregano and bake at 400
  degrees until browned and
  cooked-about 15 to 20 minutes
- While potatoes are cooking
  cook the burgers to preference
- Serve burgers over romaine
  lettuce and plate with salad and
  sweet potato wedges

Zesty Mediterranean Chicken Skillet

6 chicken thighs
Package of pre cut vegetables including onion, peppers and zucchini
2 garlic cloves crushed
Lemon juice from 2 lemons
2 tablespoons avocado oil
1 tablespoon oregano
1 tablespoon basil
1 teaspoon cumin
Sprinkle of sea salt and pepper
3 cups cooked brown rice (1 cup uncooked should yield about 3 cups cooked)
Thyme sprigs to serve

- Preheat 375 degrees
- Place thighs in oven safe skillet or baking pan and sprinkle oregano, basil, cumin salt and pepper over the thighs…coating evenly

- Add the garlic and vegetables to the oven safe skillet
- Pour over the lemon juice and avocado oil
- Bake in the oven for about 25 to 30 minutes until chicken is crispy and cooked and veggies are tender
- Serve with ½ cooked brown rice

Snack Recipes:

Baked Sweet Potato

- Prepare ahead and top with 2 tablespoons salsa or hummus

Low Sodium Soup

1 cup low sodium soup

- Choose your favorite recipe and cook up ahead of time or if short on time you can purchase store bought

Note: You can find some enzyme soup recipes under the smoothies section for homemade options

Veggies and Hummus

½ cup cut vegetables of choice
¼ cup hummus

Hummus Recipe-
1 can chickpeas (no salt added)
¼ cup tahini
¼ cup olive oil
½ cup lemon juice
3 cloves of garlic
1 teaspoon ground cumin
½ teaspoon oregano
½ teaspoon chili powder
Salt and pepper to taste

- Drain chickpeas keep ¼ cup of the liquid
- Place chickpeas and ¼ cup liquid in the food processor
- Add additional ingredients to the food processor

- Puree until smooth and creamy-
  about 2 minutes

*For a yummy variation add 1 ripe
pitted avocado and 1 cup of cilantro
leaves. YUM!

Garden Fresh Caprese:

1 heirloom tomato (or tomato of your
choice) sliced into 6 pieces
6 pieces of high quality mozzarella
cheese with no fillers
6 tablespoons of fresh pesto
6 Basil Leaves
High Quality Balsamic Vinegar (in a
glass bottle)

Assemble the tomato, cheese, pesto,
sprinkle fresh balsamic vinegar and
top with a basil leaf.

Greek Yogurt Dip and Fresh Vegetables:

Dip Ingredients:

1 cup of whole fat greek yogurt with low sugar content (Read the label to find best option…I usually use Fage)
4 garlic cloves
¼ teaspoon garlic powder
¼ teaspoon salt
2 teaspoons oregano
2 teaspoons basil
1 teaspoon ground pepper
1 teaspoon lemon or lime
1 teaspoon avocado oil or olive oil
1-2 teaspoons dill optional

Vegetables:

1 cup of fresh cut veggies of choice (I love to do cucumber, carrot and broccoli)

Mix all dip ingredients together, chop veggies of choice and enjoy! You can adjust the spices to your specific tastes. Also use as a pizza sauce, wing dip or sandwich spread. You can also add nut milk, small dash of vinegar, and feta cheese to make a delicious salad dressing!

Fresh Pineapple and Cottage Cheese:

½ cup fresh cut pineapple (or fresh fruit of choice)
½ cup cottage cheese

Enjoy!

Boiled Eggs and Blueberries

2 Medium to Hard Boiled Eggs
Salt and Pepper to Taste
½ cup blueberries or fruit of choice
Yum! Enjoy!

Egg and ½ Avocado

1 egg
½ avocado
Salsa (optional)
- Prepare egg to your liking…scrambled, hard boiled or fried
- Slice avocado
- You can add 2 tablespoons of salsa if you want to spice it up!

Note: This is a great thing to order if you have to go out to eat for breakfast! You just up it to two eggs!

Dried Fruit and Nut Mix

Purchase dried fruit (no sugar added) and nuts and mix together to make your perfect blend or make your own at home! I love to use my dehydrator and make dried bananas, mangos and strawberries and then mix with walnuts and cashews!   Serving Size is Half Cup

Apple and Nut Butter

1 apple

2 tablespoons nut butter

- Slice apple
- Spoon out 2 tablespoons of nut butter of choice
- Note: This is another great on the go snack! I use a slicer and slice the apple with the core still in the center. My friend had a great idea and she placed a rubber band around the sliced apple to keep it together with the core still in the center and then placed it in a plastic bag! You can put the nut butter in a small glass container and away you go!

Greek Yogurt Fruit and Chocolate Frozen Treats

3 cup of whole fat greek yogurt with low sugar content (Read the label to find best option…I usually use Fage)
¼ cup pur maple syrup or honey
Large handful of dark chocolate chips (about ¼ + cup)
1 ½ cups fresh fruit of choice diced into small pieces
½ teaspoon vanilla extract

- Line a baking pan or rimmed cookie sheet with parchment paper
- Mix ingredients together in large bowl
- Spread out in the pan

Fresh Nuts: Almonds, Walnuts, Pecans etc

1 cupped handful of fresh nuts of choice (should equal 10-15 nuts)

Small snack pack of Fresh Mozzarella Balls

Choose the snack pack of real fresh mozzarella! Should only include the cream and salt.

(Peanut Butter) Snack Balls

There are many variations of snack balls, but they are a perfect snack and can be modified to include your favorites. I have included the basic "oatball" recipe below with some add in options!

¾ cup nut butter (I usually use peanut butter for these)
¼ cup honey
2-3 Tablespoons water
2 cups uncooked gluten free oats

- Mix all ingredients together in mixing bowl

- Wash hands and moisten with water
- Roll into 1 inch snack balls
- Enjoy or top with your favorite items such as cocoa nibs/chips, chopped nuts, coconut flakes, dehydrated fruit etc
- Two Snack Balls Makes a Serving
- Store the remaining balls in a glass container or plastic bag in the refrigerator. You make a double batch and freeze!

A "Date" with Mango Energy Balls

2 cups pitted whole dates
1 cup raw cashews
1 cup dried mango or any other dried fruit of choice (These are yummy with dried cherries and mango together!)
2 tablespoons coconut flakes (optional)

- Place dates, cashews, and dried fruit in a food processor and blend until smooth.
- Stir in coconut flakes
- Roll into 1 inch balls and store in refrigerator or freezer

Veggies and Hummus

½ cup cut vegetables of choice
¼ cup hummus

Hummus Recipe-
1 can chickpeas (no salt added)
¼ cup tahini
¼ cup olive oil
½ cup lemon juice
3 cloves of garlic
1 teaspoon ground cumin
½ teaspoon oregano
½ teaspoon chili powder
Salt and pepper to taste

- Drain chickpeas keep ¼ cup of the liquid
- Place chickpeas and ¼ cup liquid in the food processor

- Add additional ingredients to the food processor
- Puree until smooth and creamy- about 2 minutes

*For a yummy variation add 1 ripe pitted avocado and 1 cup of cilantro leaves. YUM!

Greek Yogurt Fruit Parfait

½ cup greek yogurt
½ cup fresh fruit of choice
1 Tablespoon clean granola (I love Purely Elizabeth!)
Drizzle of Honey
- Layer the fruit and yogurt and top with granola- add a drizzle of honey on top! Enjoy!

Greek Yogurt and Dark Chocolate Chips

½ cup greek yogurt

¼ cup dark chocolate chips (70%
Cocoa or higher)
Mix and enjoy!

Roasted Chickpeas

1 15 ounce can of chickpeas with no
salt added
1 Tablespoon white vinegar
½ teaspoon cayenne pepper or space
of choice…I love Wasabi!
¼ teaspoon sea salt

- Position oven rack in upper section of oven and preheat to 400
- Mix all ingredients together with the chickpeas in a bowl
- Lightly spray a rimmed baking sheet with olive oil
- Roast the chickpeas stirring at least twice until browned. This usually takes about 30 minutes.
- Let stand and cool for 30 minutes. The chickpeas will be crisp when cooled and will stay crisp for 2 to 3 hours at room

temperature. To re crisp
remaining peas place back in
oven at 400 for 5 minutes

Banana Dippers

2 bananas cut into fourths
¼ cup melted dark chocolate or
smooth nut butter

- Dip the banana pieces in the
  chocolate leaving the top of the
  banana not dipped. Place on
  parchment paper and tray and
  place in the fridge.
- Chill in refrigerator for at least
  30 minutes before serving

Dark Chocolate Covered Fruit

1 square of HU Dark Sea Salt
Chocolate or any 70% or higher and
half a banana or ½ cup berries.

- I like to melt the chocolate and
  dip my fruit;). Or you can

choose any snack that you like from the week.

Avocado Toast

1 slice of Eziekel or Fresh Fermented Sourdough
½ avocado
1 finely chopped clove of garlic
sea salt and pepper to taste
½ teaspoon lemon juice
Garlic powder to taste preference

- Toast bread
- Cut and pit avocado
- While bread is toasting…place all other ingredients in a bowl and mash together with fork.
- Spread on toast
- You can top with any veggies or even an egg if you are eating as your breakfast!

Fruit and Almonds

½ cup fruit of choice with 5 almonds

Smoked Salmon Toast

1 slice of Eziekel or Fresh Fermented Sourdough
1 tablespoon pesto
1 ounce smoked salmon
½ teaspoon lemon juice

- Toast the bread in toaster
- Spread Pesto
- Top with Salmon
- Sprinkle Lemon Juice on Salmon
  YUM!

Dark Chocolate Cashews
1 cup unsalted cashews roasted or nut of choice
6 ounces dark chocolate 70% or higher
Pinch of flaky sea salt

- Use mini muffin tin with liner and lay out about 20 to 24 tins
- Divide cashews evenly

- Place the chocolate in a small pan and melt stirring continuously over medium-low heat with a non-stick spatula
- Spoon about 1 teaspoon of chocolate over each mini tin of cashews
- Sprinkle flaky salt evenly over each tin
- Freeze for about 3o minutes
- Store in a ziplock bag in freezer or refrigerator YUM!

Lemon Blueberry Nice Cream

3 medium ripe bananas sliced and frozen
⅓ cup lemon juice
½ teaspoon vanilla extract
¾ cup frozen blueberries

- Blend together bananas, lemon juice and vanilla extract in food processor
- Transfer to a medium bowl
- Stir in blueberries and serve- you can store in an airtight

container in the freezer for up to
1 month. I make a larger batch
and store in the freezer when I
am food prepping! You will be
glad you did! YUMMY!

Greek Yogurt Fruit and Chocolate Frozen Treats

3 Cups full fat greek yogurt
¼ cup honey
1 teaspoon vanilla extract
1 1/2 cups sliced strawberries
¼ cup mini dark chocolate chips

- Line a rimmed baking sheet with parchment paper
- Mix the yogurt, honey and and vanilla in a bowl and spread evenly onto backing sheet
- Top with strawberries and chocolate
- Freeze for at least 3 hours
- Once frozen, break into pieces, wrap in parchment paper, place

in airtight container for easy grab and go snack!

Carrot Juice or Carrots

Juice from carrots or ½ cup fresh carrots

Dark Chocolate Cashew Clusters

1 cup unsalted roasted cashews or nut of choice
6 oz dark chocolate
Pinch of flaky sea salt

- Prepare 24 mini muffin tins with liners
- Divide the nuts evenly between the tins
- Melt chocolate over medium low heat until smooth
- Spoon about 1 teaspoon of melted chocolate over each of the tins
- Sprinkle evenly with sea salt
- Freeze for at least 1 hour

- Place tins into an airtight container and enjoy your snacks!
- Eat 3 mini tins per serving

Lemon or Blueberry Lara Bar

- 1 bar of choice (read ingredients on snack bars and select ones with only real and non-processed ingredients!)

Guacamole and Baked Corn Tortilla

½ avocado

1 small clove garlic minced or you can use a tablespoon of garlic powder or everything bagel seasoning

1 tablespoon lime juice

Salt and pepper to taste

1 corn tortilla (organic) I like to make these homemade with masa, salt and water:)

½ teaspoon avocado oil

- Mix guacamole ingredients in small bowl
- Cut corn tortilla into triangles and mix up with the avocado oil
- Place on cookie sheet in the oven and bake until crisp
- Serve on a plat together and enjoy!

Open Faced Rice Cake Sandwich

1 brown rice cake
1 tablespoon almond or nut butter of choice
½ apple sliced
Sprinkle of flax or chia seeds
Pinch of cinnamon

- Spread nut butter onto rice cake
- Placed sliced apples on top
- Sprinkle with cinnamon and chia seeds

Berries and Dollop of Greek Yogurt

½ cup fresh berries of choice

Dollop of greek yogurt
- Place ½ cup berries in bowl
- Top with a dollop of greek yogurt and enjoy

Bonus Content

You want to start your journey, but you need some support! We are here to help! Below I have included a 1-week sample meal plan with meals and snacks that you can follow by referencing the recipes printed in this book! If you would like a full range of support including, interactive drop-down meal plans, menus, shopping lists, coaching, and more, please visit:

carolinasunshinewellness.com

Meal Plan	Monday	Tuesday	Wednesday	Thursday	Friday	Saturday	Sunday
Week 1	July 22	July 23	July 24	July 25	July 26	July 27	July 28
Breakfast	Mixed Berry Bliss Smoothie	Cucumber Refresher	Avocado Toast with Egg	Chai Vanilla Smoothie	2 Egg Scramble	Oatmeal Banana Pancakes	Spinach Egg Scramble & Berries
Lunch	Inflammation Buster Smoothie	Pear Salad	Veggie Beet Hummus Wrap	Mango Quinoa	White Bean Salad	Bacon Avocado Sandwich & salad	Chicken Salad Salad
Dinner	Chocolate Dinner Smoothie	Coconut Quinoa	Chicken Pesto Avocado Boats	Build Your Own Pizza	Taco Lettuce Wraps	Chicken Picatta Casserole	Sunday Night Steak Dinner
Snacks	Carrots or Carrot Juice	Veggies and greek yogurt	Greek Yogurt Fruit Parfait	2 hard boiled eggs and blueberries	Pineapple and Cottage Cheese	Berry Basil Smoothie	Choose Favorite Smoothie
	Squash or Tomatoe Soup	Cucumber, fresh basil & balsamic	Dried Fruit and Nut Mix	Strawberry Vanilla Smoothie	"Date" with Mango Energy Balls	Veggies and Hummus	Veggies and Hummus
	Optional Veggie and Salsa Snack	Yogurt, Lemon and Honey	Optional Veggie and Salsa Snack	1/2 cup sliced veggies & salsa	Handful of Nuts	"Date" with Mango Energy Balls	Hu Chocolate and Banana

I hope that you will embark and your own wellness journey and cultivate a joyful and healthy spirit!

Carolina Sunshine Wellness

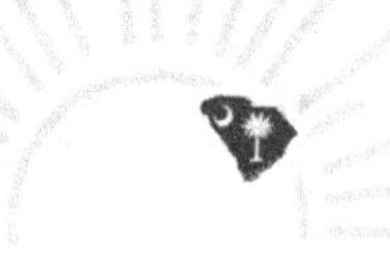

Carey and Pat Shannon
carolinasunshine@gmail.com